SHHHH SECRET

PART-2

GARRIEMA SHAH

TABLE OF CONTENTS

WHY YOU SHOULD READ THIS BOOK

By now you must have overcome the basic skin care problems of *how to get rid of unwanted pimples, how to make your skin healthy and brighter by various secret skin care kitchen recipes.* This "*recipe*" word sounds out of the box topic when we talk in regards to our skin, it sounds like you know the recipe for your favourite cuisine!

The way we humans cook food is very much similar to the way beauticians prepare facial mask, bleaching mask or toner mask and other types of concentrated chemical beauty treatments which gives short-term results. See I am not against any chemical beauty product or beauty salon, which sometimes prove to be beneficial for your skin, but they are too costly. Visiting salon once a week or in 15 days as per your budget is completely fine. I also visit salon for wax, threading and facials because sometimes we girls need pampering and a bit of relaxation from our stressful lives which only a salon can offer. So it is perfectly alright to visit beauty parlour once in 15 days or a week, solely depends on your budget. But I would not recommend facials every week, once a month is ok. Opt for a herbal facial. PLEASE AVOID - Skin whitening facials.

The need to have a more fair complexion is famous across Caribbean, African and Asian countries because of certain beauty standards set across the world. After researching the market about skin whitening products I was shocked to find out that how much adverse effect it can have on your health.

Whitening facials have lots of chemicals induced in it. Chemicals which are used in skin whitening products includes hydroquinone, mercury and steroids. Hydroquinone is a toxic chemical, it is used in rubber manufacturing and hair dyes. And this harsh chemical is present in skin whitening creams. It has bleaching properties, slows down the formation of enzyme, tyrosinase, which in turn reduces melanin produced. Hydroquinone is found to be carcinogenic, i.e. cancer causing. Some countries have imposed a ban on this chemical to be sold as a skin whitener. If we talk about another chemical, Mercury used in skin lightening products, creams containing mercury causes skin rashes, skin discolouration and even scarring.

According to World Health Organisation (WHO), using skin whitening products which have Mercury can lead to nervous system and liver damage. So the conclusion is- *if you are serious about your overall being then stop using skin whitening products.*

One major difference between chemical beauty products and natural kitchen found products is that in former case, there are 99.9% chances of getting wrinkles at an early age and various types of other beauty problems. Because there are some girls who have a very sensitive skin, which is prone to harmful chemicals, so they prefer Ayurvedic products. And nowadays there are so many Ayurvedic products being manufactured in different countries, and their price is also too high to digest. Beauty problem is solvable by use of natural products which can be easily found in your own kitchen.

Since ages India is the only country where Ayurveda has taken birth and has given many happy solution to all the people across the globe. We are not going to discuss about Ayurvedic achievements rather we are more concerned on our daily skin problems which some way or the other hinder our growth in each and every area of life.

In this book, you will get to know the amazing formula to **remove dark spots, sun tan, how to get a glowing, healthy and radiant skin and how to remove wrinkles** which can be embarrassing sometimes and it generally lowers down your self esteem especially when you have to present yourself amicably in any important event of your life. It can be your best friend's wedding, your important presentation in office or maybe your wedding or maybe even your first date! Obviously you would want to look beautifully flawless. If you are a teacher, you have to be presentable. What if a beautiful teacher have dark circle s around her eyes or patches of sun tan?

Those days were gone when students only came to school just for education but in present time, students are more attracted towards the personality of a teacher. In fact, some schools hire presentable teachers for their school's reputation. Whether you are a teacher, lawyer, banker, engineer, doctor or maybe CEO of some company, or any other profession, you have to be presentable. Being presentable doesn't necessarily mean that you have to be beautiful. Now let us clear this big difference between presentable and beautiful. If you have large eyes, well-shaped nose, protruded lips apart from plastic surgery which I never recommend to anyone. Then you are considered to be beautiful. And if you do not possess none of the above qualities but you are well dressed, outspoken personality with shiny skin then you are presentable. Who you want to be? Obviously the second one - presentable.

Lets get ready for another dose of beauty solutions for a more natural beautiful look!

"A girl should be two things, CLASSY and FABULOUS"

- Coco Chanel

CHAPTER 1. HOW TO REMOVE DARK SPOTS NATURALLY?

Are you in constant urge to remove dark spots naturally? How does it feels like when you see black spots on the face of a beautiful girl? Obviously It would look very odd. Every female has this desire of blemish free flawless skin but it is equally hard to achieve. If you use below mentioned basic home remedies then in a while you will be able to achieve your long awaited goal of getting a beautifully flawless skin. Most females find dark spots uncomfortable living with and start covering them with makeup which ultimately makes them spend lots of money on heavy priced commercial beauty products. In your surrounding markets or in tv commercials you see many companies selling variety of creams and lotions which have been labelled as ***"best dark spot removal cream"***. But there are many skin lightening creams which have bleach that is popular to make skin fair in complexion. Many folks have already suffered from skin damage or irritation as they have excessively used such creams which are easily available in market.

What is a dark spot?

In medical language, it is hyper pigmentation which results from the overproduction of melanin in your skin. This hyper pigmentation is basically caused by exposure to ultraviolet (UV) rays, ageing, use of chemical cosmetics, deficiencies of mineral and vitamins, imbalance of hormones or stress. There may be numerous reasons which could be possibly responsible for dark skin patches.

If you really want to get rid of such situation then you have easy homemade remedies that will treat the problems of dark spot naturally. In this new age generation where everyone has forgotten their roots, you can still go back to your basic roots and make the full use of ancient knowledge. It is now no more a herculean task to attain a blissful perfect flawless skin with no marks and no dark spots to hide and brood over. Transformation from dull and dark spotted skin to clean and spotless skin can be attained with the correct beauty regime without spending your fortune.

NOTE: In every remedy I have mentioned about washing face which means washing off with only plain water. DO NOT USE FACE WASH, else remedy won't work on your skin. Somewhere I have mentioned to wash off with plain water and somewhere I have not particularly mentioned plain water. So please spare me on this part as it is quite understandable to rinse off your face with plain running water. Over the internet, in some articles, blogs or posts you must have seen about washing with lukewarm water. It is not mandatory, if you wash with normal running water then also it is fine!

USEFUL HOME REMEDIES TO REMOVE DARK SPOT:

1. Lemon juice - This is one of the most easiest and quick solution to lighten the spots. Lemon is high in Vitamin C which lightens dark spots on your face. The natural acid in lemon have long been used as an organic bleaching agent to lighten dark spots. Lemon act as a natural bleaching agent that can do wonders for your skin. Citric acid found in lemon helps in breaking the melanin pigment and reduce its excessive production. Lemon remedy is very easy to follow and will cost you near to nothing in comparison to high priced treatment products in the market or prescribed by a dermatologist.

Application:

The best way to use lemon on your skin is you can apply it directly on the face. Dip the cotton ball in lemon juice and apply on your spots or you can rub lemon on your spots directly also. Continue this process for at least 2 weeks to get the desired result.

PLEASE NOTE: Do not use lemon if you have open sores or lesions on your skin. Plus avoid going out in the sun just after using the lemon juice as it can make your face photosensitive.

2. Potatoes- These are another important source of home remedy for black spots. You would have never thought the remedies to remove dark spots are present inside your fridge. **Potatoes** are natural bleaching agents which help to fade away the spots and blemishes. The starch present in potato helps in minimising the pigmentation while its enzymes promotes healthy and flawless skin.

Application:

Cut a slice of potato, place the slice directly on your black spots, patches or pigmentation. Leave it on for 5-7 minutes and then wash your face with normal water.

OR

Peel off the layer and grate a potato, add 1 tablespoon of honey and apply the mixture on your face. Leave it for 15 minutes, then rinse off with water.

OR

You can mix pinch of turmeric powder and lemon juice in equal proportion. Apply the paste on your spots. Leave it on for few minutes and rinse off with water.

3. Aloe Vera has many healing properties, Aloe Vera gel contains polysaccharides which stimulate growth of fresh skin cells to reduce dark spots.

Application:

Extract the pulp from aloe vera leaf and apply all over the face before going to bed. In the morning wash your face regularly, you will see the results immediately.

4. Sandalwood :

Sandalwood is prominently used in Indian culture as a daily ritual in prayers. It has antiseptic and germicidal properties, which helps to clear dark spots, blemishes and inhibit bacterial growth.

Application: Make a paste of sandalwood powder by adding rose water and apply all over the face. After 10-15 minutes wash off with water.

FOR DRY SKIN : Use milk instead of rose water to prepare the face mask.

5. Turmeric-

Turmeric has been used since ages for health benefits. It repairs free radical damage and reduces skin pigmentation and discolouration.

Application: Combine turmeric powder and sandalwood powder in equal quantities, add rose water to make a paste. This is the loveliest combination in giving you quick results + you will enjoy the process. Apply the mask all over the face and wash off after 15 minutes. You will see immediate effects, it will make your skin supple and smooth.

6. Vitamin E-

As dark spots are caused by vitamin deficiency and specifically Vitamin E deficiency is the main cause of dark and black spots. It is one of the easiest process to apply Vitamin E oil capsules daily.

Application: You just need Vitamin E capsule and needle, puncture the capsule with a sewing needle. Squeeze the capsule, rub the Vitamin E oil on your dark spots gently before going to bed. Wash off next day. Do it on a regular basis for instant desired results.

For oily skin I would not advise to use this method. Skip this one.

7. Milk-

Raw milk is loaded with all the nourishing nutrients for the entire body since it is not heated or pasteurised, nutrients are intact and preserved. Presence of lactic acid in milk helps in exfoliating the skin, vanishes facial skin pores and lightens dark spots.

Application: Pour raw milk into a bowl, dip a soft cloth, and wipe it all over your skin. Do this at least everyday to see results.

OR

You can use your fingertips and directly massage your skin with raw milk.

8. Castor oil-

Castor oil is extracted from the castor seeds, is an age-old remedy used by many civilisations since ancient times. It is commonly found in Africa and the Indian subcontinent, its usage is not only restricted to these two regions-it is used worldwide.

Castor oil is crammed with omega-3 fatty acids, which are the magic ingredient that helps reduce pigmentation. Omega-3 acids stimulate the growth of healthy tissue, hydrate the skin thereby giving clean and supple skin.

Application: Take 1 teaspoon of castor oil and apply on your face, massage in upward circular movements, focussing more on affected areas. After massaging for about 5-7 minutes, wash it off with a mild cleanser. Use it twice a day for better results.

PLEASE NOTE: If you have oily skin or acne, avoid using it as oil worsens these issues.

OR

Add about half a teaspoon of turmeric to a teaspoon of castor oil, you can thicken the mixture by adding more turmeric. Apply the paste onto the skin and leave it for an hour. Wash off with lukewarm water. Use it once a day.

9. Papaya-

Papaya is replenished with certain enzymes that help in diminishing dark spots and blemishes. It has natural bleaching properties to clear pigmentation. Papaya has a general usage in many skincare products. It is rich in antioxidants which includes Vitamin A, C, E and contain magnesium and potassium.

Usage of Papaya on different skin types:

DRY SKIN:

Ingredients required: Papaya, milk and almonds (should be soaked overnight)

Mix papaya and almonds equally and form a paste, add milk to the mixture. First cleanse your face with zero cost naturally homemade cleansing lotions which I have described (specific cleansing lotion for specific skin type) in part 1 of this book - Shhh Secret, Part-1.

PLEASE NOTE : If you have not read the Part- 1 of this book, then please go through Part-1 to get familiar with natural homemade face cleansing process as facial cleansing is the first step in getting a beautiful blemish free skin.

Completely clean your face with natural homemade cleanser and make sure face is properly cleansed. Apply the above mentioned paste on all over the face. Be patient for 25 minutes and wash. Please make sure your face should be semi dry before washing off the paste.

OILY SKIN:

Ingredients required: Papaya and lemon juice.

Application: Mash the papaya and mix lemon juice and form a paste. Apply this mixture to your cleansed face and leave on for about 20-30 minutes then wash off.

SENSITIVE SKIN:

Ingredients required: Papaya, honey and aloe vera.

Application: Mash the papaya properly, add honey and aloe vera gel, mix the paste and apply it evenly on the cleansed face. Leave it on for 20-30 minutes, then wash off with water.

CHAPTER 2. HOMEMADE FACE PACK RECIPES

There are certain skin types which are naturally dry and winter makes things even worse, but at times even oily skin tends to be dry and rough. Most of the people become victim to other counter remedies that doesn't necessarily work in a large number of cases, which is completely dependent on various skin types. Therefore, it is best and easy to turn towards homemade face packs for your skin without any side effect and will work definitely.

There are "n" no of reasons for skin dryness, such as:

A. Dehydration

B. Hot showers

C. Sun exposure

D. Certain medication

E. Malnutrition

F. Winter weather

Before applying face pack on your face, follow CTM techniques which have been clearly mentioned in Part-1 of this book series.

FACE PACK FOR DRY SKIN:

1. Papaya facial mask-

Papaya contains antioxidants, flavonoids, vitamin B and minerals such as potassium and magnesium that has immense benefits for the skin. Presence of Vitamin A in papaya nourishes and rejuvenates dry rough skin whereas potassium helps in hydrating skin cells and restoring moisture. If you use papaya on a regular basis then it will be icing on cake as the regular application of this fabulous fruit prevents skin ageing, wrinkles and age spots.

Take a slice of papaya, smash it well, no need to mix with any other ingredient. Apply on your face for 15 minutes the wash off with normal water.

2. Yogurt and Rosewater Pack-

Yogurt is rich in multivitamins and lactic acid. It serves as a deep moisturiser which revives dull skin. The nutrients in yogurt have effective anti-inflammatory and anti-oxidant properties and acts as a natural remedy for pigmentation and age spots. Rosewater is a natural cleanser that removes oil, sebum, impurities, dirt and dead cells.

Application: Take 2 tbsp of yogurt and add 1 tbsp of rosewater to it. Mix it well and apply on the cleansed face. Be patient for next 30 minutes and wash off with water.

3. Honey-

Honey is a natural moisturiser for skin and helps in retaining moisture and also exfoliate skin to remove dead cells.

Application: Use your fingertips and apply on your face and neck. Wash off after 30 minutes, you will see your smooth and radiant face immediately.

4. Banana & Olive oil pack-

Banana is a rich source of antioxidants, it acts as a nourishing natural remedy to treat dry, rough and dull skin.

Application: Mash one ripe banana to form a smooth paste, add 1 tablespoon of olive oil to it, mix well and apply on clean face. Wait for 20 minutes and wash off thoroughly with water. It is advised to repeat the this procedure 2-3 times per week to get naturally blemish free skin.

5. Aloe Vera & Cucumber Pack-

Aloe vera gel is a promising nourishing and hydrating agent helps in retaining moisture while Cucumber is 95% water, it also helps in maintaining skin moisture and hydrates dry skin to make it soft, smooth and supple.

Application: Squeeze out gel from aloe vera leaf, add some grated cucumber and mix the ingredients. Apply on face and other dried areas. Stay for 30 minutes and rinse off. Use this remedy 2-3 times a week.

FACE PACK FOR OILY SKIN:

1. Tomato, Honey and Cucumber-

Cucumber is rich in potassium, magnesium, Vitamin A and E which is a cure for oily skin. Tomatoes are powerful astringent agent which reduce excess oil from surface of skin which makes it as a great treatment for oily skin.

Application: Extract the juice of cucumber and tomato, add 1 tbsp of honey to the mixture and mix it well. Apply the mask on your face evenly, wait for 25 minutes, then rinse off with plain water.

2. Lemon juice and Honey-

We all are familiar with lemon juice properties, it is rich in Vitamin C which makes your skin healthy and glowing. On the other hand Honey has great rejuvenating properties which makes your skin supple.

Application: Mix 1 tablespoon of honey and lemon juice well. Apply the paste on cleansed face, massage gently for few minutes. Wait for 20-25 minutes then wash off with plain water.

3. Apple and Honey-

Honey is a very good moisturiser for oily skin, it also reduces skin infection. Apple has cooling astringent properties which lowers excessive oils by minimising skin pores.

Application: Grate the apple into finer pieces, add honey and mix the paste well. Now apply the pack on your face evenly, after 20-25 minutes, wash off with lukewarm water.

4. Rose Water and Multani Mitti(Fullers Earth)-

Fullers Earth is a very powerful home remedy for reducing excessive oil of the face. It has amazing astringent properties and helps in minimising size of the pores and makes skin smoother. And rose water maintains the pH balance of the skin.

Application: Add 2 tbsp of Fullers Earth's powder in a glass plate, add rose water and make equal amount of mixture. Make a smooth paste out of it and evenly apply on the clean face & neck. Wait for 25 minutes, then wash off with plain water. Repeat this remedy twice a week for best results.

5. Lemon juice and Potato Pack-

Lemon and potato juice both act as natural bleaching properties. Potatoes are a rich source of potassium, calcium, proteins, Vitamin A and C.

Application: Peel off potato and grate it into finer pieces. Extract the juice from potato. Mix it equally with lemon juice. Apply the pack on clean face and neck. Wait for 30 minutes and clean with plain water. Repeat this remedy for thrice a week for desired results.

6. Orange, Honey and Banana Face pack-

This is the ideal face pack for oily skin. Banana helps in wiping out the excess oil.

Application: Mash the ripe banana, fresh honey and orange juice in a blender equally. Paste will be formed and apply it on your face, after 15 minutes rinse off.

CHAPTER 3. HOW TO VANISH EARLY SIGNS OF AGEING - FINE LINES AND WRINKLES

Everyone of us wants to live young and die young, nobody wants to age. Very well said "life begins at 40!" But by 40 how many of us stay young physically? Not mentally or emotionally I guess! But physically. Your physical body tends to age with time. Your hair greys out, some of you develop fine lines and wrinkles. These are basic signs of ageing, which is a natural phenomena of human body. But whenever you look into the mirror you tend to deny all these signs. Many times you have seen beautiful celebrities in glossy magazines, newspaper, movies and you must have envied that actors in their 40s look so young and stunning. And you are an old rag still in your 30s! See I am not trying to bog you down or break your heart but I am here to help you out. This is the basic reality which we need to address and sort it out in a best possible way. And this is the only sole reason I have started writing book series on beauty solutions in a much lesser cost effective way without any side effects.

Cause and effect theory exist everywhere, if there is a cause, then effect will follow.

Causes:

Root cause for wrinkles to appear on a face is a result of lot many facial expressions, overexposure to sun, smoking, lack of water intake, medications and some of the environmental factors. All over the world people spend billions of dollars on expensive treatments, laser surgeries, botox and so many to remove or delay the ageing process. Many of these treatments claim but have no effect while others may have some mediocre effect or a considerable amount of success.

As we human beings get older, our skin becomes more thinner, drier and looses elasticity which leads to wrinkles and fine lines on the skin. There are other lifestyle and environmental factors responsible for a toll on your physical appearance which includes lack of sleep, chronic stress, sun damage, pollution and smoking.

These were the general causes which leads to develop wrinkles and fine lines. One of the major factor which I personally feel is responsible to develop fine lines is worrying. Yes we worry a lot, those worries can be fear of losing a job, or partner, maybe you have insecurities about your relationship, worries of not paying your bills, and the list goes on and on. There is no end and you cannot either put a full stop to your worries. Huuuuuuh! Now what to do? How to stop worrying?

See I am not here to give you philosophical lectures on being positive, radiating positive vibrations. We all are very much familiar with the law of attraction, science has made this very clear. So instead of worrying on petty issues, start thinking on how to overcome all your problems. When you eat healthy, think healthy, then definitely outcome will be healthy results.

So spare out some time for your anti-ageing process and please stop buying wrinkle free products. Here are some quick-to-use remedies for reducing wrinkles:

1. Milk powder + Honey-

 Milk powder is easily available in any store, it makes skin softer and nourishes the skin. Honey gives a natural glow on your face. Mix 2 tbsp of honey, warm water and milk powder, mix them equally without forming lumps. Apply on your face evenly, wait for 10 minutes. Wash it off thoroughly.

As I have mentioned in the first part of Secret series that natural beautification is a slow and gradual process. At least be patient for minimum 2 weeks, but you need to be consistent on your efforts. Alternate day you can apply some of the remedies depending on your routine.

2. Green tea-

Detoxification of skin is the most essential part of any skin regime. As possible try and have green tea regularly, it gifts you with a fresh skin and wrinkle free skin too. If you are subservient to your taste buds then you can add 1-2 tbsp of honey into the green tea, then you can have it with a sweet taste.

3. Aloe Vera-

Importance of Aloe Vera has been again and again stated till this part of the series. Keep one thing in mind - ***Aloe Vera is a nectar for your all beauty problems***. It contains *malic acid* which improves elasticity of your skin thereby reducing wrinkles.

Application: Extract Aloe Vera juice from the leaf and apply it all over the face, if you can resist then wash your face in the next morning. You will see the difference.

Do you know the most beautiful aspect of applying homemade kitchen recipes on your face? You feel that your skin is breathing, yes that always happens with me whenever I apply homemade recipes. And Aloe vera is the bestest part of my beauty regime. I want you to apply as much Aloe Vera as you can whenever you are at home. In 4 days only you will see the magic!

4. Banana + Honey-

Bananaaassssss....yeah it sounds yuck but it serves as a beautiful shock to your skin. Banana is famously named as "Mother Nature's Botox", it contains loads of nutrients which delays the ageing process and reduces wrinkles and fine lines.

Application: Mash 1 ripe banana, add 1 tbsp of honey, mix the paste well. Apply evenly on your face, wait for half an hour then rinse off.

Banana comprises of 75% water which hydrates the skin and leads to younger looking skin.

5. Vitamin E-

Vitamin E is a very good moisturiser, it is rich in antioxidants and has anti-inflammatory and photo protective effects on the skin which reduces skin's vigour and vanishes wrinkles.

Application: Extract the oil from Vitamin E capsule as per your requirement. Apply this oil on your face and surrounding areas and massage in circular motions for a few minutes. Leave on for few hours or you may sleep and wash off your face with normal water the next morning. You can do this therapy regularly before going to bed.

I remember the day when I tried mixing Aloe vera gel with Vitamin E capsule. I just applied the paste on all over my face and neck(recommended). In the morning I was super excited that I will get double effects but to my surprise there was least affect on my face. I went on deep and realised that I need to use this remedy one by one as I used to do earlier. Till today I cannot understand why both these super foods for skin didn't work wonders for my skin.

Anyways I would advise you all to not mix these 2 mixtures. Day 1 apply aloe vera and wash off next morning and Day 2 apply Vitamin E capsule and wash off next morning. After washing off do not use any chemical products, whatever natural remedies you have prepared, go ahead with it.

6. Argan oil + Castor oil-

Castor oil is very good in production of elastin and collagen in the skin, which as a result vanishes fine lines at a certain period of time. On the other hand Argan oil contains fatty acids and Vitamin E that replenishes the skin.

Application: Mix both the oils in equal quantities and massage on the affected area. Leave it on for rest of the night.

People who have oily or pimple prone skin avoid using this remedy. You can skip to other remedies mentioned.

CHAPTER 4. HOW TO GET RID OF DARK CIRCLES

Dark circles under the eyes is one of the defect in your beauty. And there are "n" no of reasons responsible, some of them are listed below:

a. Oversleeping

b. Sleep deprivation

c. Skin irritants in cosmetics

d. Exposure to sun

e. Alcohol

f. Allergy

g. Sickness

h. Hormonal Changes

i. Stress

Please focus only on homemade remedies to lighten the dark circles. With time it will vanish, please be consistent in your efforts.

Getting rid of dark circles in few easy methods:

1. Rose Water-

Without any doubt rose water is one of the simplest technique to get rid of dark circles.

Dip cotton balls in rose water and put onto your eyes and relax for an hour. After removing the cotton pads, you will feel stress free and relaxed. Rose water will lighten the skin under eyes.

2. Aloe Vera-

Aloe Vera gel when applied under the eyes, it soothes and protects the skin.

3. Cucumber-

Cucumber is one of my favourite remedy to treat dark circles and puffy eyes. It really works wonder for your eyes as it completely removes the dark circles as the under skin of eyes is very light and one cannot afford to use harsh ingredient onto that skin. So cucumber is perfect for under eye treatment. You can use cucumber slices or juice to reduce dark circles and refresh the eye area.

4. Tomato-

Using tomato under eyes is one of the most effective remedies to treat dark circles. Slightly rub the tomato slice under your eyes to lighten and brighten the skin.

It is a multipurpose effective ingredient, you can use it all over the face and neck to tone your skin. In one stroke 2 purpose will be solved- one, removing dark circles; two, toning the skin.

5. Almond oil-

Almond oil has anti-inflammatory and antioxidant properties and contains Vitamin E, Vitamin K, retinol which helps to smooth delicate skin under your eyes.

Before laying down for bed, Gently massage oil under your eyes for few minutes. For oily skin avoid this remedy skip to other remedies.

6. Coconut oil-

Coconut oil contains high fatty acids which reduce inflammation and improve circulation. It is great in skin strengthening and is a very good antioxidant.

Before going to bed massage coconut oil in circular movements, next morning whole oil would be soaked up into your skin. Within 4-5 days you will see the difference.

Please Note: Make sure you do a patch test of coconut oil on your skin as some people have reported allergies to coconut oil.

There are other remedies too which exist, like chemical peels, Vitamin C serum which your skin specialist might suggest. More advisable if you follow home remedies, it will add Natural Vitamin C, minerals, proteins and other vitamins into your skin.

After going through these remedies for dark circles you might be wondering "Oh man, I know some of the remedies, I want a shortcut.....to my dark circles......I have to be perfect for my first date. Tomorrow is my friend's wedding!" For wedding and immediate occasions, you can always go ahead with a herbal or Ayurvedic concealer. Herbal or Ayurvedic is any which ways effective without zero side effects. Effective in the sense it does not harm your skin like any other chemical cosmetics or products. Whenever you buy any beauty product always and always go through the contents behind the bottle. Do not just blindly trust the brand because you have seen your favourite celebrity endorsing that very same brand!

I have been through the most impatient problems in which I just wanted result overnight. Remember nothing comes handy and there is a no shortcut for any kind of success. You have to work

hard and consistently keep putting your efforts then only you
will be able to achieve the desired results.

CHAPTER 5. HOW TO REMOVE SUN TAN

Who doesn't love summers? They can be so much fun! Having sun bath on the beaches with beautiful bikinis on the hot body, or simply having fun with friends in a warm and sunny weather. As a result, you develop a tanned skin. After few days of flaunting your tanned body you want to remove the tan as soon as possible.

When itching or burning sensation happens, then it can ruin your summers too!

Lets quickly get through some easy to use sun tan removing recipes:

1. Honey & Papaya-

Papaya is such a beneficial ingredient for skin that its enzymes has been used in skin whitening and exfoliating products. Honey makes skin soft and supple. Combination of these products prepare an effective sun tan removal recipe.

Application: Mash 1/2 ripe papaya and add 1 tbsp honey, mix it well and apply evenly on the tan affected areas. Leave it on for half an hour then rinse off thoroughly.

2. Aloe Vera + Fullers Earth + Rose Water-

Fullers Earth(Multani Mitti) is a favourite beauty remedy from time immemorial. It will soothe your sun burns and cleanses your skin thoroughly and stimulates circulation. By now you are very much familiar with the properties of Aloe Vera and yes it is a very good suntan removal gel. About rose water is that it will help in making a efficient paste.

Application: Mix aloe vera gel, Fullers Earth and Rose water in equal proportion. Form a paste and apply on affected areas. After 10-15 minutes, wash off.

3. Tomato-

Tomato is famous for its depigmentation properties, with regular usage it will help to get rid of tan. It is one of the easiest and fastest remedy to remove suntan.

Application: Squeeze out the juice from refrigerated tomato and apply it on the affected areas. Leave it on for 30 minutes then wash off. Tomato can be applied daily for quick removal.

4. Milk-

The presence of lactic acid in milk helps in fading away sun tan in few days plus it will evens your skin tone and helps in nourishing your dry and dehydrated skin.

A word of caution: if you are allergic to milk, then do not use this remedy. Skip onto next in whichever method you are comfortable with.

5. Lemon + Sugar-

The Lemon Juice is a popular sun tanning agent! Sugar is an amazing exfoliant, erases the dead and dark skin cells and other dirt as well.

Application: Make a paste of sugar and lemon juice equally, use it as a scrub on affected areas. Massage it gently in circular movements depending on your massaging capacity. Continue this for 3-4 minutes then rinse off thoroughly.

Use this scrub every alternate day to get rid of sun tan.

6. Cucumber-

Cucumber is a very good coolant, it calms down irritated, inflamed skin and refreshes and rejuvenates the skin ultimately leading to lightening of the tan.

Application: Add honey to the extracted cucumber juice, make a paste and apply it on the sunburnt areas for 20 minutes. Rinse with cool water. Repeat this process daily.

7. Wheat Flour-

Selenium present in wheat exhibits antioxidant properties that help to fight free radicals and helps in protecting your skin from harmful UV rays. Vitamins, Zinc and minerals present in wheat promotes collagen production and improve skin texture.

Application: Make a thick paste of wheat flour and water and apply on the tanned areas. Wait for 15-20 minutes then rinse off. You can repeat this process daily for effective immediate results.

These were the easy, quick to use effective homemade remedies for suntan removal. However there are many more complicated homemade remedies for sun tan which I have not mentioned over here. As I said my main mission is to bring out the easiest best possible methods to overcome common beauty problems. So the above mentioned methods are good enough to remove suntan from your face and other affected areas.

CHAPTER 6. HOW TO DEVELOP A GLOWING, HEALTHY AND RADIANT SKIN IN JUST 4 WEEKS

Now I am sure that you have learnt the art of naturally cleansing, toning, moisturising and removing all sorts of debris from your skin. So, now get ready for a radiant and spectacular glorifying beauty in just 4 weeks! Yes, it is possible and that too naturally without using any chemical products. The only condition is that you have to apply various recipes regularly then only you will be able to achieve your desired goal of getting beautifully flawless skin in just 4 weeks. And the mixtures and paste which have been mentioned are very simple and easy to use to give maximum benefit in a lesser time.

Apart from externally using the household remedies there are many healthy options to try out for making skin more clean and healthy by intake of various diet. To be more precise, I have not mentioned the kind of food intake for healthy and glowing skin as everybody is well aware of the right kind of foods for our better well being. Rather I have stressed out more on making and using right recipes for your natural beauty.

1. Baking Soda-

This recipe is one of the most easiest and quickest homemade remedy for a radiant skin. Baking Soda is a natural exfoliator and cleanser. It contains anti-bacterial and anti-fungal properties.

Benefits: It absorbs excess oil from the skin and provide oil-free complexion and prevents production of melanin that causes skin darkening. It also stops acne/pimples from developing. Baking soda facial exfoliator removes black/white heads which are deep seated inside your pores.

Application: Add 1 teaspoon of baking soda and water, mix it well to form a paste. Apply it evenly on your face and neck*(both parts are recommended in every session of beauty therapy)* Wash off after 6-7 minutes.

2. Turmeric-

Turmeric is rich in antiseptic, anti-bacterial and anti-inflammatory properties. There are many other procedures to make a turmeric paste but here I have mentioned the most easiest method for application.

Benefits: Turmeric is a great natural exfoliator and helps in removing dead skin cells. It improves skin's texture and protects skin from rashes, redness and infections.

Application: Mix 2 teaspoons of lemon juice and 1 teaspoon of turmeric and form a paste. Apply it evenly and after 15 minutes wash off with water. If possible use this remedy at night twice a week.

3. Coconut oil-

Coconut oil is naturally antibacterial, anti fungal, moisturising and as per research, great for atopic dermatitis.

Benefits: It is a very good moisturiser for face as well as for flaky lips.

Application: Simply massage the coconut oil before going to bed as during whole night your skin will absorb the coconut oil completely.

Oily skin people avoid this method.

4. Aloe Vera-

By now you must be familiar with the amazing qualities of Aloe Vera. By regular usage of aloe Vera gel it is confirmed that your skin will attain a perfect radiant glow in just 2 weeks!

5. Lemon-

It is a very good astringent, rich in Vitamin C and antioxidants. The most amazing quality of lemon is it removes dead skin cells and gives a glowing skin.

Application: Mix in equal quantities of mashed tomatoes and lemon juice. Apply it on your face. Leave it to dry completely. Wash off throughly.

Benefits: This remedy will bring immediate glow to the face and removes skin's blemishes, lightens the skin and make it supple.

6. Papaya-

Presence of potassium in papaya hydrates the skin and removes dullness. Special enzyme present in papaya is "papain" which removes dead cells and other impurities.

Application: Add 3-5 tbsp of papaya with 1 tbsp of honey. Mix it well and spread the mask all over your face and leave on for 10-15 minutes. Afterwards wash off with water.

Benefits: Papaya is a natural beauty enhancer because of its exfoliating, whitening and healing properties.

7. Milk+ Honey+Gram Flour+Turmeric+Sandalwood powder-

Mixture of above ingredients is most popularly known as "ubtan" In India. This is the one and only golden homemade remedy to get a flawless and radiant glow on your entire body. It is an auspicious traditional remedy for Indian brides and grooms before their D-day for glowing skin. Ubtan can be used by anyone for any occasion to get a healthy beautiful glow naturally.

Benefits: Nowadays it is very popular so it is available as pre-made combo packs. However it is very easy to make "ubtan" at home to get the best desired results for glowing, clear and lighter skin. This remedy can be applied on your face and body to get maximum better results for your overall beauty.

Various types of "Ubtan" Pack for face and body:

A. Gram Flour+RawMilk

This is one of the easiest and basic "ubtan" and can be done thrice a week for instant results in a much convenient way.

Application: Combine the above 2 ingredients to make a good paste. Apply this paste, avoid talking and lay down for 20-30 minutes. Afterwards wash off throughly with plain water

B. Gram Flour+Honey+Turmeric powder+Sandalwood powder+Raw milk

This is the main course "ubtan" which is used by brides and grooms before their marriage.

Application: Take equal amount of above mentioned ingredients depending upon your usage. Apply the well mixed paste on your face and body, wait for 30 minutes, then wash off with plain water. Because of turmeric's presence you may develop yellowish skin, don't worry, wait for 2 days it will vanish. Make sure do not use any kind of face wash just after the "ubtan". And don't bother yourself about the leftovers, you can refrigerate it and use it whenever required.

So these were my personally used tips and tricks to get a healthy, flawless, even skin tone and radiant skin. I really wanted to share my beautiful journey and *"being beautiful"* experiences with all the beautiful girls inside out. Please trust me if you use at least some of the mentioned instant tips on your skin then I guarantee you will get a desired beautiful skin. But you have to be consistent in your efforts, there is no leave and no laid back approach in beauty regime. This is the time you have to be really serious about healthy skin care routines. It doesn't matter of what age or what complexion you are, what matters is your sincerity towards achieving your goal.

Best of Luck in your beauty journey! For any queries, concerns, questions or any issues, please leave a comment on my blog- www.buzzobia.com. I would be happy to guide you in your beauty journey!

About The Author

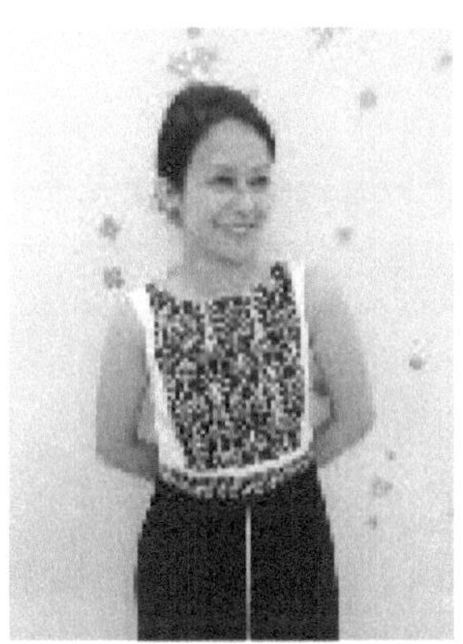

GARRIEMA SHAH is the Amazon author of 2 fiction books - *U Love me, Love is you* and 2 non-fiction books - *Shhh Secret-1 and Shhh Secret-3*. This is the *Part-2* of *Secret series*. She lives in Mumbai, India. Garriema loves educating and inspiring people in all over the globe about her experiences and observations. Right now she is on a mission to bring awareness about natural beauty regime.

Other Books By Garriema:

1. U Love me?

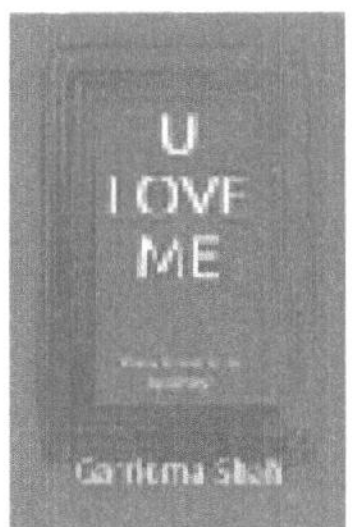

2. Love is You

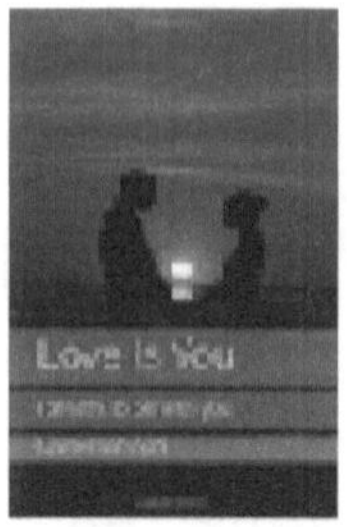

3. Shhhh Secret- Part-1

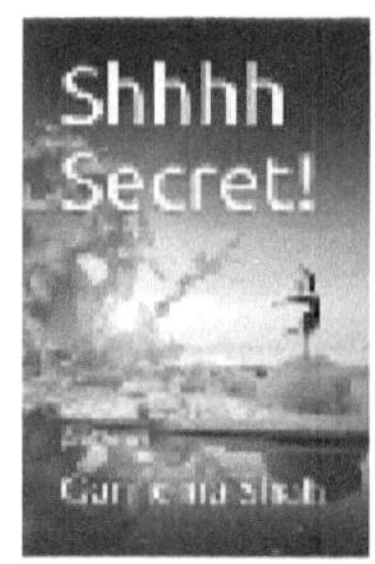

4. Shhh secret Part-3

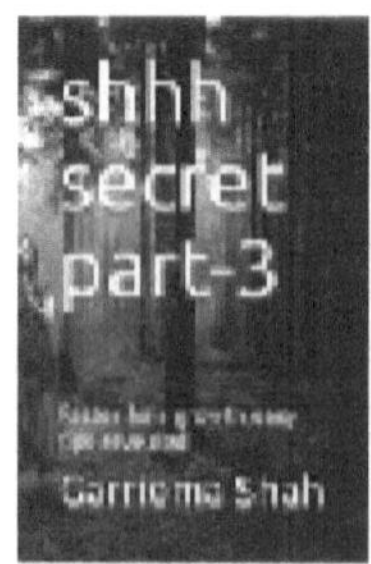

ONE LAST THING...

If you enjoyed reading this useful piece of information or want any changes, I'd be very grateful if you'd post a short review on Amazon. Your support really does make a difference as I really want genuine feedback and reviews. And I read all the reviews personally so I can get your feedback and make this book even better.

Thanks again for your amazing support!